Frequently Asked Questions

all about
MSM

MARGARET DENNISON, MA

AVERY PUBLISHING GROUP
Garden City Park • New York

The information contained in this book is based upon the research and personal and professional experiences of the author. It is not intended as a substitute for consulting with your physician or other health care provider. Any attempt to diagnose and treat an illness should be done under the direction of a health care professional.

The publisher does not advocate the use of any particular health care protocol, but believes the information in this book should be available to the public. The publisher and author are not responsible for any adverse effects or consequences resulting from the use of any of the suggestions, preparations, or procedures discussed in this book. Should the reader have any questions concerning the appropriateness of any procedure or preparation mentioned, the author and the publisher strongly suggest consulting a professional health care advisor.

Series cover designer: Eric Macaluso
Cover image courtesy of Barry Axelrod Studios

Avery Publishing Group, Inc.
120 Old Broadway, Garden City Park, NY 11040
1-800-548-5757 or visit us at www.averypublishing.com

ISBN: 0-89529-970-4

Copyright © 1999 by Margaret Dennison, M.A.

All rights reserved. No part of this publication may be reproduced, stored in a retrieval system, or transmitted, in any form or by any means, electronic, mechanical, photocopying, recording or otherwise, without the prior written permission of the copyright owner.

Printed in the United States of America

10   9   8   7   6   5   4   3   2   1

Contents

Introduction, 5

1. MSM—A Sulfur Compound, 7

2. MSM for Beauty, 21

3. MSM for the Treatment of Allergies, 31

4. MSM and the Digestive System, 41

5. MSM for Aches, Pains, and
   Other Ailments, 53

6. Using MSM, 63

Conclusion, 71

Glossary, 73

References, 77

Suggested Readings, 89

Index, 91

Introduction

Imagine a product that enhances your overall beauty by making your hair shiny and your nails strong, while it minimizes your allergic reactions to foods, animals, dust, and pollen. Next, envision a product that relieves the pain and inflammation of arthritis, stiff joints, and many other painful musculoskeletal conditions, and also alleviates constipation and stomach acidity. Now, imagine that all these benefits are available in a single supplement. Does this sound too good to be true? Well, the incredible news is that this remarkable product really does exist, and it is available at your local health food store.

Though it may surprise you, the natural product that can do all these wonderful things is sulfur. No, not the odorous, inorganic sulfur like that found in hot springs, toxic smog, and the vapors of volcanoes, but the organic version of sulfur that is known as methyl-sulfonyl-methane, or MSM for short. In case you didn't know, sulfur is present in every cell of your body, and is an important constituent of your skin, hair, and nails. It's also the main ingredient in collagen—the connective tissue that holds your body together—and is an essential component of several amino acids. What's more, your body depends upon an adequate supply of this mineral for a healthy acid/alkaline balance, which is essential to life. This is why supplementing with MSM is such a good idea.

In *All About MSM*, you'll learn about this newly discovered supplement and how it can enhance your beauty and improve specific health conditions, such as arthritis, diabetes, and asthma. You'll also learn how it can counteract the effects of a sulfur-deficient diet. Most important, you'll learn exactly how you can put this supplement to work for you so that it can naturally and effectively improve your health and appearance.

1.

MSM—A Sulfur Compound

Although sulfur has existed in the earth's crust for millions of years, its use as a nutritional supplement is quite recent. Methyl-sulfonyl-methane, or MSM as it is commonly called, is an excellent supplemental source of sulfur. This naturally occurring organic sulfur compound is found in the tissues and fluids of all plants, animals, and humans. MSM supplements are virtually nontoxic and pose none of the risks associated with other supplemental sources of sulfur. Considering that MSM is pretty new to the supplement market, it's not surprising that there are many questions to be answered regarding this remarkable product.

Q. Where does MSM come from?

A. MSM is the natural result of a series of events that begin when simple forms of marine life, such as algae and plankton, take in inorganic sulfur and convert it into organic sulfur compounds, known as dimethylsulfonium salts. The ocean water then transforms these salts into a new compound known as dimethyl sulfide (DMS), which is released as a gas into the upper atmosphere. There, in the presence of ultraviolet light and ozone, DMS is converted into dimethyl sulfoxide (DMSO), which in turn is oxidized into MSM. When it rains, these sulfur compounds are returned to the earth, where plants absorb them through their root system and incorporate MSM into their structure. Animals eat the plants and take MSM into their bodies. We eat both the plants and animals, thereby taking in the sulfur we need for our bodies to function properly. Eventually these sulfur compounds are returned to the ocean and the cycle starts over.

Q. How were the therapeutic effects of MSM discovered?

A. The medical application of MSM was discovered by Stanley Jacob, MD, of the Oregon Health Sciences University in Portland, Oregon, and his associate, Robert Herschler, a research chemist for a paper manufacturing company. This discovery grew out of their pioneering research into the therapeutic abilities of dimethylsulfoxide (DMSO), which is produced in abundant quantities as a by-product of the paper milling process. In the course of their research, Jacob and Herschler concluded that MSM is the main healing element in DMSO.

Q. Why should I use MSM instead of DMSO?

A. Although DMSO is effective for a wide range of conditions, it causes some unpleasant side effects, such as reddening and itching of the skin, nasal congestion, shortness of breath, excess intestinal gas, and allergic reactions. DMSO also has a strong sulfur odor, resulting in a garlicky smell when taken orally or applied externally to the body. None of these side effects are dangerous, merely unpleasant. However, one property of DMSO does give cause for concern: when it is applied externally, it acts as a powerful carrier for other substances, including toxic ones. These substances are carried into the body through the skin and mucous membranes, where they may do damage. The presence of possible manufacturing impurities in DMSO is another cause for concern. For this reason, the DMSO available from commercial outlets is manufactured mainly for industrial and animal use, and should not be used by humans except with great care.

Both DMSO and MSM are powerful painkillers and anti-inflammatories. But MSM is a much better choice because it is safe and odorless, and does not result in any of the adverse reactions shown by DMSO. Supplementing with MSM is a safe way to supply your body with the sulfur it needs to function at its best.

Q. What is sulfur, and why does my body need it?

A. Sulfur is an acid-forming mineral that is part of the chemical structure of several amino acids. Your need for sulfur is clear when you consider that it is found in every cell of the body and that it is an important substance in the creation and regeneration of the body's tissues. Sulfur must be present for collagen to be produced, making it a vital component in the formation of cartilage and connective tissues. The major amino acids, vitamins, antioxidants, and hormones that are essential to the healthy functioning of your body all contain sulfur. Sulfur helps to form the keratin that is required for healthy, strong hair and nails. And without sulfur, the acid/alkaline balance of the body cannot be maintained. In fact, although sulfur has not been given much recognition, it is the fourth most abundant mineral in the body.

Q. How important are minerals to the body?

A. You probably already know that you must get an adequate supply of vitamins in your diet for good health. But you may not know that getting an adequate supply of minerals is just as essential. Because minerals play an important role in accelerating the chemical processes in your body, a lack of necessary minerals can be dangerous to your health.

The mineral content of various foods depends upon many factors, such as geologic conditions, the state of the soil, the effects of acid rain, and the consequences of overprocessing. Of the total nutrients your body needs, only 0.3 percent are minerals. This may seem like an insignificant amount, but without this small percentage, the remaining nutrients cannot be properly utilized. Sulfur is just one of a whole collection of minerals without which your body cannot function properly.

Q. What are good food sources of sulfur?

A. Beef, poultry, fish, milk—particularly unpasteurized milk—and eggs are all good food sources of sulfur. Soybeans, turnips, dried beans, Brussels sprouts, and kale are also good sources. Some other vegetables, such as broccoli, cabbage, garlic, and onions, contain small amounts of sulfur. You should note that the small quantities of sulfur that are present in vegetables are largely destroyed during the cooking process.

Q. Do I get enough sulfur in my diet?

A. Chances are that your diet does not provide you with enough sulfur. Like all minerals, sulfur cannot be manufactured by the body, so you must get this nutrient from outside sources. Normally, sulfur is passed on to you through the foods you consume, such as plants that have absorbed sulfur from the soil and animals that have eaten these plants. However, these plants are only as nutritious as the soil they grow in, and unfortunately, the use of chemical pesticides and fertilizers in modern factory farming contributes to the massive depletion of natural resources in the soil. Therefore, conventional food sources may no longer be an adequate source of sulfur.

An additional cause for the lack of natural sulfur is our culture's dependency on processed foods, which are even more deficient in sulfur than fresh foods. So it's a good idea to compensate for this lack of natural sulfur through supplements. MSM is a safe way to do this.

Q. What happens if my body doesn't get enough sulfur?

A. Several things can happen. Your body may not be able to repair or replace damaged tissue quickly enough. When this occurs, the body compensates by producing abnormal cells that may lead to disease and illness. You may also experience a heightened sensitivity to pain since the presence of adequate sulfur balances the buildup of pressure in the body's cells. The healthy acid/alkaline balance of the body may also be compromised, and this, in turn, may make you susceptible to disease, and may prevent the body from turning food into the energy needed to fuel its functions.

Sulfur deficiencies are also associated with gastrointestinal problems, a poorly functioning immune system, arthritis and rheumatism, acne, and memory loss. Allergies may become more extreme. A deficiency can also lead to brittle nails and hair, dry skin, and dermatological problems.

Q. What compounds in my body depend on sulfur?

A. Sulfur is contained in many compounds essential to your body's functions. For example, glutathione—the body's primary antioxidant—requires sulfur to effectively combat free radicals. Like all antioxidants, glutathione prevents or slows the oxidation process caused by reactions with oxygen. In so doing, it helps to neutralize the effects of free radicals, thereby lowering your risk of cancer, heart disease, and other illnesses.

Glucosamine also depends on sulfur from glucose and glutamine for its production. This compound plays an integral role in the formation of ligaments, tendons, and other membranes, and makes cartilage strong, healthy, and resilient. Biotin, a B vitamin essential to the production of fatty acids, also requires sulfur. Other sulfur-dependent compounds include fibrinogen, a blood-clotting agent; insulin, a hormone that balances the body's glucose supply; and thiamin (vitamin

B_1), a primary factor in the metabolism of carbohydrates. And the list goes on.

Q. What are amino acids and which ones contain sulfur?

A. Amino acids are the building blocks of proteins. Without amino acids and the proteins that they constitute, your body would be unable to create muscle, ligaments, tendons, organs, glands, nails, hair, and many vital fluids. There are twenty-eight known amino acids of which eight are "essential," meaning that you must get them from your diet because your body cannot produce them. The essential amino acids are histidine, isoleucine, leucine, lysine, tryptophan, valine, phenylalanine, threonine, and methionine. Your body uses methionine to synthesize three other amino acids—cysteine, cystine, and taurine—which together are known as the sulfur amino acids. While the sulfur amino acids are very important for good health, all of the amino acids—essential and non-essential—must be present to ensure a fully functioning body. They work so closely with one another that if only one is absent, the others cannot be utilized and protein synthesis cannot take place. Without protein, growth ceases and all bodily functions break down.

Q. What do the sulfur amino acids do?

A. The sulfur amino acids all play important roles in good health. For instance, methionine assists in the breakdown of fats, helps to detoxify harmful toxins, and is required for the formation of DNA and RNA—the carriers of genetic information; cysteine has many medical uses, such as acting as a detoxifier for the treatment of drug overdoses, and helps to raise the levels of T-cells, which are white blood cells central to the efficient functioning of the immune system; and taurine is a component of bile—a digestive juice produced by the liver and stored in the gallbladder that is used in breaking down fatty foods and controlling cholesterol.

Q. If I eat foods rich in these sulfur amino acids, why should I bother taking MSM?

A. A balanced diet of organic foods goes a long way toward meeting your body's needs. However, as mentioned previously, our soil is so depleted of nutrients that there is no longer any guarantee that you will receive all of the necessary nutrients from the food you eat. That's why it's a good idea to supplement your diet with MSM to ensure that your body is getting all the sulfur that it needs to function at optimal levels.

Q. Is sulfur the same as sulfa drugs and sulfites?

A. Definitely not. Organic sulfur is a nutrient and, as you learned, a necessary part of natural chemical processes in the body. It is not to be confused with sulfa-based drugs or sulfites, which are forms of inorganic sulfur. Sulfa-based drugs are synthetic, meaning that they do not occur naturally. They are used for the same purposes as antibiotics, and, in some people, can cause strong allergic reactions.

As for sulfites, not only do they have no nutritional value, but they destroy certain vitamins in the body, and may cause nausea and diarrhea. Despite these negative effects, sulfites are used as preservatives in food, and may appear on a food label under the names of sulfur dioxide, potassium bisulfite, sodium sulfite, or sodium bisulfite.

2.

MSM for Beauty

When you think of beauty products, do your thoughts rush to those delicate creams you massage into your face to remove wrinkles overnight? Since we live in a world of quick fixes, it's understandable that we expect to scoop instant beauty from a jar. We want results, and we want them now. However, the instant external results we get from these products tend not to last. Maintaining healthy skin is also an inside job. No lotion or cream can do for us what good nutrition coupled with an adequate mineral and vitamin intake can. This chapter will explain why MSM is an essential contributor to our natural beauty, from the inside out.

Q. How will MSM affect the appearance of my skin?

A. MSM acts to keep the skin's cells and tissue soft. Keeping the skin soft ensures that it remains elastic enough to allow stretching and movement without damage. Smooth, flexible skin is less prone to wrinkles and dry flakiness, not to mention stretch marks. (Though stretch marks are usually associated with pregnancy, they can occur anywhere on the body that the skin does not have enough elasticity to expand.) So, in a nutshell, MSM helps to keep you looking young by keeping your skin smooth and supple.

Q. What else does MSM do for my skin?

A. Plenty. Skin is your largest organ, which means that it also provides the largest area for the release of toxins from your body in the form of sweat. Although fewer toxins will be produced with proper nutrition, it is still inevitable that some toxins will find their way into your body. MSM facilitates the removal of these toxins. The softness, flexibility, and permeability of your skin that result from taking MSM make it easier for sweat to escape, and thereby release toxins from your body. It's important to avoid developing hard or leathery skin because these conditions prevent sweat from escaping through the pores, resulting in a buildup of toxins in your body. But with MSM supplements, rough skin shouldn't be a cause for concern.

Q. What happens if sweat glands become clogged?

A. Different sweat glands have different functions, and depending on their location in the body, they excrete water, salts, or other bodily waste. If any of these glands become clogged, they cannot process waste matter.

When this happens, toxins back up in the body, leaving a fertile breeding ground for bacteria, which can then can move in and cause illness. Poor nutrition can also lead to clogged pores and sweat glands, so in addition to taking MSM, you should eat a healthy, well-balanced diet.

Q. Can MSM help teenagers who suffer from acne?

A. Studies have shown that the severity of acne that has been triggered by the raging hormones of puberty can be reduced with MSM. Common teenage acne is usually the result of clogged pores most likely due to overactive oil glands. By keeping the skin soft, flexible, and permeable, some of the excess oil can escape, avoiding bacteria buildup in the pores. In addition, a body that does not have a healthy acid/alkaline balance is more susceptible to acne-causing bacteria, and as you have learned MSM helps your body maintain a healthy acid/alkaline balance.

Q. Exactly how does MSM work to keep my skin elastic?

A. For your skin to be healthy and elastic, its layers must be connected so that they can work together and support each other. The main component of connective tissue is collagen, and sulfur is needed by the body to produce collagen. Sulfur forms the disulfide bonds that are necessary to hold tissue together. Collagen works with a protein known as elastin, which gives the skin its elasticity. The presence of sulfur also prevents collagen from cross-linking, meaning that it prevents it from forming undesirable bonds with other proteins or lipids, which may result in dry or hard skin.

To understand the importance of connective tissue, it is helpful to consider the various layers that comprise your skin. The first three layers are known collectively as the *epidermis*. They constantly throw off dead cells, which rise to the surface of the skin, and are then renewed from a deeper layer of the epidermis. Underneath the epidermis is another layer called the *dermis*, containing blood vessels, sebaceous glands, sweat glands, and hair follicles. A layer of fat known as the *subcutis* makes up the bottom layer. Each of these layers perform different functions and have different structures.

Q. Why is collagen so important?

A. Collagen—the single most common protein in the body—is the main component of skin and bones. The tough, fibrous, and insoluble nature of collagen enables it to hold the connective tissues of the body together. Without collagen, the body would collapse in a shapeless heap.

In our youth-oriented society, we hear a lot about collagen as the great rejuvenator. This substance has been injected under the skin to reduce wrinkles and to create a more youthful appearance. But because natural chemical processes in the body break down the injected collagen, its effects last for only about two years. Drugstore shelves also display an impressive array of collagen-containing beauty products, but like injected collagen, the collagen in these beauty products has temporary results. That's why it is important to make sure that the body produces enough natural collagen with healthy chemical links so that its needs are supplied from within. Since sulfur is vital for this process, supplementing with MSM is a great way to ensure that your body has the opportunity to produce enough collagen. You should also note that vitamin C is a major component of collagen, and the importance of getting adequate amounts of this vitamin in your diet can hardly be overstated.

Q. How does MSM help hair to become healthier and nails to become stronger?

A. Sulfur helps the body to form keratin, the protein that makes up the main part of the outermost layers of your hair and nails. It is a tough, fibrous protein that is very resilient to the effects of damaging chemicals and other harmful agents. Each strand of hair has its own keratin supply, which is stored at the root. Since you have many thousands of single hairs on your head, you can well imagine what a constant, abundant supply of keratin is necessary to constantly feed your hair. MSM can help provide your body with the sulfur it needs to maintain your keratin supply.

Sulfur is also contained in biotin, a B vitamin that is essential for shiny hair and strong nails. You may be interested to know that the natural inclination of hair to be straight or curly is maintained in part by the sulfur amino acids.

Q. Since MSM is so beneficial to skin, hair, and nails, is it the only beauty treatment I need?

A. Unfortunately it's not quite as simple as that. While MSM is essential for a healthy body with lustrous hair, clear skin, and strong nails, it does not act alone. The human body requires many minerals, vitamins, and other nutrients that work as a team to produce a vibrant, disease-free environment. The key here is balance. Although MSM helps to strengthen nails, soft nails can just as easily be caused by lack of vitamin A. Similarly, limp or lifeless hair may have causes other than a lack of sulfur. That's why it is important to follow a nutritious diet and to make sure that you are taking in and absorbing enough of all the essential vitamins and minerals. If your diet is less than healthy, you may need to augment it with other vitamin and mineral supplements.

3.

MSM for the Treatment of Allergies

Are you one of the people who sniffle and sneeze their way through the allergy season and back off in panic when the neighbor's cat drops by for a visit? In the midst of your misery, it may be poor consolation to know that you are not alone. In fact, an estimated 40 million people in the United States suffer from allergies. However, you will be happy to know that there is now a natural solution. Studies have shown that MSM is effective in reducing reactions to many common allergens. In this chapter, you will learn about allergies and their causes, and how MSM works with your body to increase your resistance to allergens, thus making your life more bearable.

Q. What are allergies and why do they happen?

A. Allergies are reactions set off by a breakdown in the normal functioning of the body's immune system. When this happens, a varied range of symptoms are manifested, including sneezing, runny nose, watery eyes, headaches, and sleepiness. Other allergic reactions include hives, stomachache, and sore throat.

Normally, the immune system acts to fight off bacteria, viruses, and other substances that cause disease, illness, and discomfort. Sometimes even ordinary substances are perceived by the body to be harmful, causing the immune system to react abnormally. The immune system goes into fight mode and produces antibodies to combat these substances, or allergens. The allergic reactions arise when the allergens bond with antibodies, releasing histamines—the substances responsible for setting off the common allergic reactions described above. Each time the body encounters an allergen, it will recall its initial reaction to the allergen and will react similarly, though the severity of the allergic reaction may vary.

Q. What types of substances cause allergies?

A. Allergens—substances that the body perceives as harmful—can include dust mites; animal dander; pollen; certain drugs; and environmental substances, such as smoke, exhaust fumes, pesticides, and other chemicals. Some people are allergic to certain foods, such as milk, wheat, or seafood. Some people are even allergic to smells, such as certain perfumes, and may react to them with a headache and watery eyes.

Surprisingly, the most common allergen is not pollen but house dust. The real culprits in house dust are the millions of microscopic dust mites that live alongside you in your home. Mites themselves are not aggressive, and it is not mite bites that spark off the allergy, but a protein that is contained in their feces. Regardless of season or temperature, mites are constantly breeding and multiplying. Since they feed off the dead skin cells that your body is continuously discarding, dust mites have an abundant source of nourishment. Once hatched from their eggs, they reach maturity within three to four weeks. They are at home in warm, cozy environments, such as blankets, pillows, carpets, and even stuffed toys. There is no way to completely get rid of mites since they thrive in normal living environments. However, you may notice a decrease in allergic reactions if you replace wall-to-wall carpeting with hardwood floors and thereby reduce the mites' living space. Also, keeping the humidity in your living environment below 50 percent can help since humidity is an important factor in the mites' survival.

Q. Can anyone develop allergies?

A. Yes, allergies can be triggered at any time during your lifetime. Just because you have never suffered from an allergy does not mean that you won't react strongly to this year's pollen or the chemicals in the new office carpet. If there is a history of allergies in your family, you may have a genetic tendency to develop them. In all cases, the severity of symptoms will depend upon your level of resistance to the particular allergen that your body is fighting. However, if that all sounds discouraging, remember that you don't have to wait for allergies to strike. Instead, you can take preventive measures by making sure that your body is getting enough sulfur, which can be accomplished by taking MSM supplements, so that the chances of an allergic reaction are minimized.

Q. How does MSM deal with allergies?

A. MSM goes straight to the cause of allergic reactions. An allergic reaction is brought on by a specific protein molecule, whose role it is to combat substances that have infiltrated the body and that the body perceives as hostile. As you learned earlier, one of the effects of MSM is that it softens the skin. It does this by softening the walls of the body's cells, which are then more easily penetrated, allowing enemy substances to be flushed out. Flushing these allergens out of the body eliminates the need for the body to react allergically to get rid of them. This process cannot happen when the cell walls are hard and impenetrable. Additionally, MSM prevents allergic reactions by coating the gastrointestinal tract in a way that makes allergen bonding impossible.

Q. How does this differ from conventional treatments for allergies?

A. Allergies are most commonly treated with various drugs. The main purpose of these drugs is to suppress allergic symptoms. So although your nose stops running and your eyes stop tearing, the reaction itself has not been addressed. Also, as with any type of synthetic drug, there is always the risk of undesirable side effects from your allergy medication.

Antihistamines are a normal treatment for allergic reactions, but they are sedatives—substances that causes drowsiness. They may help you get a good night's sleep without scratching and sneezing, but it's extremely dangerous to take them if you must drive, operate machinery, or do anything that requires your full attention. Hence, this treatment limits the scope of your activities and interferes with your ability to perform your regular duties.

Another conventional form of treatment is

allergy shots. However, it can be a long process before the doctor is able to determine exactly what substances your body is reacting to. Once that's established, the allergy shot will protect you only against that particular allergen, and will offer you no protection against other substances to which you may develop an allergy. Immunotherapy treats allergies by giving increasing doses of the allergen over an extended period of time, so as to stimulate the body to produce antibodies that will eventually block allergic reactions. About two-thirds of the people treated with immunotherapy react favorably. However, immunotherapy treatments can require anywhere from two to three years to take full effect. For allergic rashes and skin conditions, a corticosteroid cream can be applied topically, but when used continuously, this cream may cause damage to your skin.

It is impossible to live in our society without being exposed to a multitude of allergens. Conventional remedies are, at best, tedious and lengthy and, at worst, dangerous and damaging. It's better to take preventive measures that include supplying your body with enough MSM, so that you can minimize the risk of allergic reactions and eliminate the need for any medical intervention.

Q. Does MSM help with all types of allergies?

A. Since MSM is acting at the level of the cause by strengthening the body's natural cleansing abilities, it is an effective means of combating all types of allergies. Research has shown that daily doses of MSM have substantially increased resistance to environmental, food, or drug allergens. Results ranged from substantial relief to complete disappearance of symptoms. There are also reports that MSM reduces allergies to some everyday, over-the-counter drugs.

Occasionally allergies may be so severe that they require conventional treatment. In these cases, MSM can be taken as an adjunct therapy. For example, additional daily doses of MSM have enabled allergy-induced asthma sufferers to reduce their amount of conventional medication by up to three-quarters. A woman who suffered from regular asthma attacks observed a radical decrease in the frequency of her attacks after taking MSM in powder form on a daily basis. Another person reported that when he took MSM in combination with vitamin C, he experienced a strengthened immune system, which in turn increased his body's ability to get rid of the allergens before he experienced an allergic reaction.

4.

MSM and the Digestive System

Taking good care of your outer appearance, such as by bathing and by brushing your teeth, is probably a regular part of your daily routine. But have you ever thought of cleaning yourself from the inside? You may think that the inside of your body takes care of itself, but in truth, it doesn't. It's been said that most diseases begin in the intestines because of lack of proper cleansing and elimination. In order for your body to process nutrients effectively, your digestive system must be in good working order. It's important to be sure that there are no foreign bodies, such as parasites, lurking about in your intestinal tract, causing damage. In this chapter, you will learn a little bit about what's going on in your stomach and intestines and how MSM can help you to clean it all up.

Q. What are parasites?

A. Parasites are animals, plants, or microbes that live inside or on another organism, known as the host, and feed off it without contributing anything to the health or well-being of the host organism. Parasites suck energy from their host without killing it.

There are many types of parasites that can infect humans, including lice, mites, leeches, ticks, and worms. They can range in size from microscopic to 30 feet in length.

Foreign foods may contain parasites that our bodies are not familiar with. Some unpleasant effects from parasite infestation that have been experienced by world travelers are known as "Montezuma's Revenge" or "Delhi Belly." These are forms of acute stomach and intestinal upsets that are characterized by diarrhea and vomiting.

Some parasites attach to the body's inner surfaces while some live in the blood, such as those parasites that cause malaria. Parasites' eggs can nest in our bedding or towels, and are ready and willing to take up residence in our bodies as soon as an opportunity presents itself.

Fortunately, MSM has been shown to help prevent parasites from attaching to the walls of the intestines. This will be explained in more detail further on in this chapter.

Q. Why do we have parasites in our super-hygienic society?

A. We associate parasites with underdeveloped countries and unhygienic living conditions. However, we no longer live in an isolated land, protected from the illnesses and diseases prevalent in other parts of the globe. In earlier times, our world was largely limited to our local area, our daily contacts were with people who grew up and lived near us, we nourished ourselves with food that was produced locally, and the world outside our community hardly affected us.

But times have changed. The increase in international travel, both for business and pleasure, means that our lives are increasingly impacted by global considerations. Each time a traveler returns from abroad, there is a good chance that he or she is transporting not only souvenirs, but some unwelcome intestinal guests. Growing international trade means that more and more exotic produce and foods are imported from foreign countries. These foods can be bearers of parasites, too.

There are many sources of parasites close to home, as well, such as in human waste or in heavy chemicals that may contaminate our drinking water supplies. These can be the sources of hookworms and threadworms. Another rich source of parasites is soil that has been contaminated by animal feces. In addition, red meat can harbor a parasite known as roundworm. For this reason among others, it is important to always wash your hands after handling raw meat of any kind. There are plenty of places where people come together in closed, restricted environments that are ideal traveling areas for parasites, such as nursing homes, day-care centers, convalescent homes, and social clubs. Also, it's possible that many household pets carry parasites, which can be passed on to their owners.

Q. How do I know if I have parasites?

A. There is no accurate way of knowing whether you are harboring parasites in your intestines or indeed in any other part of your body. The reason for this is that parasites can cause symptoms similar to many common medical conditions. Since parasites are hard to identify, parasite infestation is often misdiagnosed. Symptoms attributable to parasites can resemble those for hypoglycemia, depression, and chronic fatigue syndrome, among many other diseases and disorders. There are tests available, including saliva tests, that can eliminate the possibility of parasites, but in general they are difficult to detect. The discovery of parasites is made more complicated by the fact that they often lie low for long periods, at which time they cannot be detected through testing. Furthermore, tests designed to locate intestinal parasites will not find parasites in your blood. Chances are that many Americans are harboring parasites, and you may be one of them.

Q. What are the effects of parasitic infestation, and how does MSM help?

A. The presence of parasites can lead to low energy, gastrointestinal disturbances, itching, and muscle pains for which there are no obvious reasons. These creatures can wreak havoc on your insides. Since they are living beings and need nourishment, they feed off your blood and tissue, and eat the nutrients that your body needs. Thus, they deprive you of the full benefit of the food you are ingesting. Parasites can continue this attack for years without detection since the symptoms they cause are so similar to those of many common ailments.

MSM has proven to be a very effective treatment for parasites. Research shows that MSM works by laying a coating over the intestinal areas where some types of parasites normally attach themselves. This coating makes it impossible for parasites to attach themselves to your body. Since they are not attached to your body, the parasites are simply flushed out of your system through the process of elimination. As an internal remedy, MSM can be used against worms, giardia, trichomonas, and other types of parasites.

External parasitic infections that show up as skin conditions, such as ringworm or athlete's foot, can be treated successfully with MSM cream. If you do not want to touch those areas for fear of spreading the parasites, MSM spray is a good alternative.

Conventional cures for parasites are usually strong drugs that have unpleasant side effects. Moreover, parasites can be elusive and difficult to treat by conventional means because of their life cycles. They may lie low for many days, months, or years, during which time you may assume that they have finally taken their leave of your body, only to find that you experience an unexpected recurrence some time later. You never know what will trigger the parasites in your body to become active again.

Making sure that you have an adequate daily intake of MSM can help to ensure that the parasites do not have a chance to make themselves at home inside your body.

Q. What else is going on in inside of me that MSM might clean up?

A. MSM is effective in treating some forms

of gastrointestinal dysfunction, such as constipation and heartburn. Perhaps you are taking in enough nutrients, but they are not being properly processed by your digestive system. MSM can help your body to better utilize the nutrients in the food you eat. MSM can also improve tolerance to food allergens. The coating that MSM puts on the gastrointestinal walls that wards off parasites also prevents food allergens from causing damage.

Q. What is constipation, and how can taking MSM help?

A. Constipation is characterized by hard, painful stools, sometimes accompanied by bleeding. This condition occurs when waste material moves too slowly through the large intestines. In dosages of 500 mg per day, MSM has been shown to bring prompt relief for chronic constipation. In addition to MSM supplementation, adding fiber to your diet can also help with constipation. Fiber is the indigestible part of many fruits and vegetables, which provides the bulk that the muscles of the large intestine need to propel waste matter through the intestines on its way out of your body. For best results, increase the quantity of fiber in your diet gradually to allow your body to get used to it, otherwise you may experience some gas and bloating. Eating prunes is also a good way to help relieve constipation.

Q. What is heartburn, and how does MSM help?

A. Stomach acid is used by the body to break down food during digestion. The stomach lining releases a form of acid known as hydrochloric acid, which is necessary for the digestion of proteins. If the valve regulating the flow of food into the stomach does not close properly, stomach acid can back up into the esophagus, causing a burning pain in the upper chest or throat area, known as heart-burn. This particular disorder can also be caused by rich, spicy foods; alcohol; or over-eating.

MSM has been shown to be more effective than the standard treatments for stomach acid. Standard treatment for heartburn involves the use of antacids and other products that neutralize hydrochloric acid. These may give temporary relief by counteracting the effects of hydrochloric acid, but a reduction in hydrochloric acid content can in turn lead to indigestion and poor absorption of nutrients. In addition, overuse of antacids can destroy the body's natural acid/alkaline balance. As you learned earlier, this can impair the body's normal metabolism. MSM helps the body maintain its acid/alkaline balance, while neutralizing the excess stomach acid. In test subjects given MSM, antacids and other products were no longer necessary or could be significantly reduced.

Q. Can MSM help with all digestive complaints?

A. MSM won't help all digestive complaints. Sometimes sluggish digestion results from the inadequate production of hydrochloric acid, in which case taking MSM would be counterproductive since it blocks the production of hydrochloric acid. Such a condition is common in older people because the body's production of hydrochloric acid slows with age. If you have this condition and still wish to take MSM to relieve other conditions or simply to enhance your overall health, it is advisable to also take betaine hydrochloride, which provides additional hydrochloric acid. Betaine hydrochloride can be found at your local health food store.

5.

MSM for Aches, Pains, and Other Ailments

The legendary reputation of the mineral baths of Europe is based on the curative powers of their sulfur-rich waters. Thousands of people visit these baths every year to find relief from their aches and pains. It's no wonder that sulfur is considered such a versatile supplement! In the 1970s, sulfur in the form of DMSO was approved for use in treatment of bladder infections. It was also used for many other painful conditions such as arthritis, gout, and bronchitis. With the discovery of MSM and its greater safety, sulfur has come out of the closet and is now more available to the general public. This chapter will take a look at some of the everyday applications of MSM in the relief of aches, pains, and other ailments.

Q. How does MSM help to alleviate pain?

A. As you learned in Chapter 2, one of the beneficial effects of MSM is smoother skin, which is the result of more supple, permeable cell walls. When the body's cell walls are supple, fluids can easily pass out of the cell, resulting in equalized pressure inside and outside the cell. In many cases, it is the difference of pressure that causes pain and inflammation. By equalizing the pressure, MSM helps to reduce pain and inflammation. Furthermore, just as permeable cell walls allow substances to flow easily out of the cell, they also allow nutrients to enter the cell with greater ease so that your body's needs are better met and your overall health is improved.

Q. Can MSM help with painful conditions like arthritis?

A. MSM brings effective relief to arthritis sufferers not by dulling the nerves so that the pain cannot be felt, but by mending some of the damage that causes arthritic pain. The two main forms of arthritis are rheumatoid arthritis and osteoarthritis, both of which can affect any of the joints including the fingers, toes, knees, neck, hips, and spine. Both conditions cause pain, stiffness, and, sometimes, complete deformation of the joint. Osteoarthritis usually affects one joint at a time, gradually destroying the cartilage. Rheumatoid arthritis, on the other hand, attacks the whole body at once and is accompanied by swelling.

The existence of adequate cartilage is necessary for healthy joints. Cartilage is a protective layer between the bones of a joint, which acts as a cushion to prevent the bones from rubbing together. It also works like a sponge to hold the fluid that provides joint lubrication and mobility. Once the protective padding that cartilage provides is gone, friction between the bones occurs, leading to painful, stiff joints. As we get older, the cartilage is not so readily replaced by the body, leaving the joints more susceptible to arthritis.

Q. What is the usual treatment for arthritis?

A. The conventional treatment for arthritis is nonsteroidal anti-inflammatory drugs (NSAIDs) such as ibuprofen or naprosyn, but they only provide temporary relief. NSAIDs inhibit the production of prostaglandin, a hormonelike substance that triggers inflammation, fever, and pain. Like many other synthetic drugs, they can have unpleasant side effects and can cause stomach upset or stomach bleeding.

Studies have shown that glucosamine, a sulfur-dependent compound, which plays an important role in the formation of ligaments, tendons, and other membranes, is more effective in the treatment of arthritis than NSAIDs. Not only does glucosamine have no side effects, but it reduces inflammation and contributes to the growth of new cartilage. As you learned earlier, cartilage is composed mainly of collagen, which needs sulfur to be produced. So taking MSM supplements along with glucosamine can enhance the health benefits of glucosamine.

Q. How does MSM help to alleviate muscle pain and stiffness?

A. Supple cell walls more easily allow unwanted substances to pass through them to be excreted from the body as waste. You are probably familiar with the muscle stiffness and cramping that can occur after a strenuous workout or sometimes even when you do an everyday activity that you are not used to doing. This stiffness is caused by a buildup of lactic acid in the cells. The cell flexibility experienced by taking MSM allows the lactic acid to pass through and be discarded, so that the stiffness does not occur in the first place. For this reason, MSM is an important addition to any athlete's supplement regimen.

A buildup of lactic acid after strenuous exercise is merely uncomfortable and will disappear. But a buildup of toxins in your body can cause illness and disease. The permeable cell walls created by MSM allow the body to release the toxins so that they do not back up inside you. This is another way that MSM contributes to your overall health.

Q. Can MSM help in the treatment of cancer?

A. Although human studies have not yet

been conducted, other studies suggest that MSM may prove to be beneficial in slowing the growth rates of cancerous tumors. A study conducted at the Department of Surgery at the Ohio State University College of Medicine showed that MSM can reduce the growth rate of colon cancer in laboratory animals. Researchers observed the effects of MSM on rats that had been subjected to harmful substances associated with colon cancer. After a two-month period, results showed that the onset of tumors was significantly slower in the animals treated with MSM than in the control group. Similar research examined the effects of MSM on breast cancer in laboratory animals and showed that though the actual incidence of tumors was not statistically affected, there was an increase in the length of time it took for tumors to appear. Furthermore, the animals did not experience any toxic reactions or significant weight loss.

Q. Can people with diabetes benefit from taking MSM?

A. MSM has been shown to be effective in the treatment of diabetes, which occurs when the body produces or uses insulin inefficiently. Sulfur is an important component of insulin, a hormone produced in the pancreas to metabolize carbohydrates. Without sulfur, the body cannot produce enough insulin, leading to excess blood sugar, so MSM may be an especially important supplement to include in your diet if you have diabetes. However, if you have diabetes, please take MSM under the supervision of a health-care professional.

Q. What other ailments does MSM help?

A. There are also many reports of dramatic results from using MSM in other areas of healing. MSM is reported to increase stamina and alertness in patients suffering from emphysema and lung tumors. It has been shown to be effective in the healing of severe burns. Severe scar tissue from burns and multiple skin grafts were treated with MSM cream, and the scarred tissue slowly transformed into healthy skin. This healing took place many years after the original injury.

MSM has also proven to be extremely effective in the treatment of asthma, easing breathing after only a few days, even in long-time sufferers. Even many years after the onset of arthritis symptoms and years of excruciating pain, MSM promoted the rapid healing of painful joints. Results were seen within a few days. Similarly dramatic results have been seen in the use of MSM for fibromyalgia. MSM has also been used in eye drops for soothing relief from eye inflammation, itching, redness, and infections such as conjunctivitis. Though these are impressive reports, in many cases the beneficial effects lasted only as long as MSM was being taken.

As soon as use of MSM stopped, the symptoms returned.

6.

Using MSM

If you suffer from any of the problems mentioned in this book, or if MSM sounds as if it could enhance your health, then you may want to try MSM to alleviate some of your ailments or simply to experience its health-enhancing abilities. All you need to do is visit your local health food store and pick up one of the readily available forms of MSM. This chapter will give you some information about usage and dosage so you can start putting MSM to work for you.

Q. How much MSM does my body need?

A. The recommended daily allowance for MSM has not yet been established. The amount you need depends on how much sulfur is already present in your body, the amount that you take in through food, your body's ability to process the mineral, and the severity of your symptoms if you are taking MSM for a specific condition. One thing is clear, however—a separate MSM supplement is necessary because it will not be included in your regular multivitamin and multimineral supplements. As you get older, it is even more important to supplement your diet with MSM, since supplies in the body become depleted with increasing age.

Q. What is the recommended dosage of MSM?

A. Stanley Jacob, MD, states that dosages of MSM can range from 1 to 2 g per day all the way up to 80 g daily. He recommends a general dosage of 1 to 3 g per day. If you find that such a small dosage is not taking effect after a week or two, you can experiment with increasing the dosage until you notice results. Any MSM that your body does not need will be eliminated naturally. MSM is nontoxic; however, as with all nutritional supplements, it is wise to have your doctor or other health-care professional monitor dosages over 10 g.

Experience has shown that a single dose is not effective. The usual recommendation is to take MSM several times during the day or over a number of days. If you feel you need a larger dose, it is best to break down the dose into several parts and take it over the course of the day, and always with meals. Studies show that in some instances, you can expect to see changes within a few days, but certainly after about three weeks.

Q. What forms of MSM are available for internal use?

A. For internal use, MSM is available as a powder or as capsules. Both of these forms should be taken with meals—not on an empty stomach. MSM powder is water soluble and can be mixed with liquid. It dissolves more quickly and readily in warm liquids so you may want to heat the water slightly or at least use it at room temperature, rather than straight from the refrigerator. MSM powder has a slightly bitter taste and may be more palatable if mixed with fruit or vegetable juice.

Q. What forms of MSM are available for external use?

A. For external use, MSM comes in lotion form. This is useful for topical treatment of inflamed areas, sore joints or muscles, or for skin conditions such as eczema. Often it is enriched with skin moisturizers. Additionally, MSM is available as a spray that can be used on parts of the body that are too sensitive to touch, such as rashes or minor burns. MSM spray is the best form to use for the treatment of external fungus, such as athlete's foot or ringworm, in order to avoid spreading the fungus by touching the affected area. MSM eye drops are available for the relief of eye inflammation, such as conjunctivitis, or to alleviate redness There is even an MSM toothpaste that can help with inflamed or bleeding gums.

Q. What should I keep in mind when I'm buying MSM?

A. When purchasing MSM in any form, make sure that there is a batch number on the bottle so that you can refer back to it if there is any problem with the product. Also check for the manufacturer's address so that you can contact them if you need to.

No matter what form of MSM you purchase, the usual precautions apply, such as making sure that the seal on the bottle has not been broken or tampered with.

Q. How safe is MSM?

A. MSM is very safe. In fact, common table salt is reportedly more toxic than MSM. Stanley Jacob, MD, states that MSM demonstrates similar toxicity to water—which means you don't need to worry about taking too much of this supplement. Your body will only extract the amount of MSM that it needs. While it is clear that MSM is essential for health, it has not yet been approved as a nutritional supplement by the Food and Drug Administration (FDA). In the meantime, MSM is available in various forms at health food stores as an over-the-counter supplement.

In several years of use and observation,

there have been no reports of adverse reactions. It is safe to take MSM in conjunction with medication. Although MSM is extremely safe, if you are pregnant or lactating, it is best to avoid all supplements and medications unless they are recommended by a health-care professional.

Q. Can I give MSM to my pets?

A. Use of MSM can enhance overall health in your pets. Horse trainers give MSM to their racehorses before races to prevent the buildup of lactic acid in muscles, which causes stiffness and cramps after exercising. Due to its anti-inflammatory properties, they also use it to treat joint pain in their horses.

You may never have thought of using beauty products on your pets, but as a side effect of being treated with MSM, they will acquire attractive, glossy coats, and strong toenails. You can add 1 to 3 g of MSM to your dog, cat, or even your guinea pig's food, as a daily tonic and/or as an aid in treating the ailments mentioned in this book.

Conclusion

By now you should understand the important health benefits of MSM. This amazing supplement can help alleviate a variety of complaints. It's also an important constituent of amino acids, collagen, and keratin, all of which are essential for a fully functioning body. MSM has positive side effects, such as glossy hair and strong nails. Furthermore, it is the most effective way to counteract the effects of a sulfur-deficient diet. As more research is conducted, and more and more benefits are brought to light, MSM will get the recognition it deserves. However, as with any nutritional supplement, MSM is not meant to be your only source of nutrients. Its purpose is to supplement a healthy, balanced diet, not to replace one. If you are abusing your body, no amount of supplements will make it function properly. Drink lots of clean water and maintain a healthy lifestyle with good food and plenty of sleep and relaxation, and the addition of MSM will further enhance your health and well-being.

Glossary

Allergens. Substances that provoke an allergic response in some people.

Amino acids. The building blocks of protein.

Antioxidant. A substance that slows oxidation and helps to defend against free radicals.

Collagen. A protein used to make the connective tissue that holds the body together.

Free radical. A molecule with an unpaired electron that causes damage to cells by stealing away an electron, which can lead to illnesses, such as heart disease or cancer.

Insulin. A hormone produced in the pancreas that metabolizes sugars.

Metabolic processes. Various chemical and physical processes that enable food to be utilized by the body, and which provide energy for vital functions.

Minerals. A group of inorganic elements essential to human health. They are also basic components of the earth's crust.

Parasite. An animal, plant, or microbe that lives in or on another organism and obtains nourishment from it without contributing anything in return.

Protein. The basic elements of all animal and vegetable tissue.

Prostaglandin. Hormonelike substance that can trigger inflammation, fever, and pain.

Sulfa drugs. Synthetic drugs used as antibiotics to fight bacterial infections.

Sulfites. Preservatives and additives used in food to prevent decay and discoloration.

Synthetic substance. A substance that does not occur naturally or is synthesized in a laboratory.

References

Baker, DH, "Utilization of Isomers and Analogs of Amino Acids and Other Sulfur-Containing Compounds," *Progress in Food Nutrition Science* (1986).

Bartfeld, IJ, Goldstein, A, "Cell-mediated Immunity: Its Modulation by Dimethylsulfoxide," *Ann. N. Y. Acad. Sci.* (1975).

Bigazzi, Pierluigi E, "Autoimmunity and Heavy Metals," *Lupus* 3 (1994):449–453.

Braverman, MD, Eric R, and Pfeiffer, MD, PhD, Carl C, *The Healing Nutrients Within*. New Canaan, CN: Keats Publishing, Inc., 1987.

Ceconi C et al.; Mol, J; "The Role of Glutathione Status in the Protection Against Ischaemic and Reperfusion Damage: Effects of N-acetyl cysteine," *Cell Cardiol* (1988).

Childs, S. J., "Dimethylsulfone (DSMO2) in the Treatment of Interstitial Cystitis." *Urol. Clin. North Am.* (1994).

Cook, Alison, "Unwelcome Guest, Reluctant Host," *Texas Monthly* (1985).

Cooper, A, "Biochemistry of Sulfur-containing Amino Acids," *Ann. Rev. Biochem.* (1983).

D'Ambrosia, E, Casa, B, Bompani, R, Scali, M, "Glucosamine Sulphate: A Controlled Clinical Investigation in Arthosis," *Pharmatherapeutica* (1981).

Dausch, PhD, Judith G, and Nixon, MD, Daniel W, "Garlic: A Review of Its Relationship to Malignant Disease," *Preventative Medicine* (1990).

Dennis, AJ and Wilson, HE, "Altered Mitogenic Responsiveness of Chronic Leukemic Lymphocytes and Normal Human Lymphocytes Treated With Dimethylsulfoxide," *Ann. N. Y. Acad. Sci.* (1975).

DiCyan, E, *A Beginner's Introduction to Trace Minerals,* Keats Publishing, New Canaan, CT, 1984.

"Earth Matters," Issue #30, Friends of the Earth, London, 1996.

Ensminger, Audrey H, et al., *Foods and Nutrition Encyclopedia.* Clovis, CA, Pegasus Press, 1983.

Gaull, GE, "Taurine as a Conditionally Essential Nutrient in Man," *Jrn. Am. Coll. Nutr.* (1986).

Hanson, RR, "Will Medicine Keep Your Horse Sound?" *The Horse* (1996).

Hendler, S, *The Doctor's Vitamin and Mineral Encyclopedia,* Fireside, NY, 1991.

Herschler, RJ, "MSM: A Nutrient for the Horse," *Eq. Vet. Data* (1986).

Herschler, RJ, "Methysulfonylmethane and Methods of Use," United States Patent 4,296,130: 1981.

Herschler, RJ, "Methysulfonylmethane and Compositions Comprising It," United States Patent 4,616,039: 1986.

Herschler, RJ, "Dietary and Pharmaceutical uses of Methysulfonylmethane and Compositions Comprising It," United States Patent 4,512,421: 1985.

Herschler, RJ, "Dietary and Pharmaceutical uses of Methysulfonylmethane and Compositions Comprising It," United States Patent 4,514,421: 1985.

Jacob, SW, "The Current Status of MSM in Medicine," *Am. Acad. Med. Prev.* (1983).

Jacob, SW and Herschler RJ, "Introductory Remarks: Dimethylsulfoxide After Twenty Years," *Annual New York Academy of Science* (1983).

Jensen, B, *Empty Harvest*, Avery Publishing Group, Inc., Garden City Park, NY, 1990.

Kharasch, N, Thyagarajan, BS, "Structural Basis for Biological Activities of Dimethylsulfoxide," *Annual New York Academy of Science* (1983).

Klein, HA, Samant, S, Herz, BL, Pearlman, HS, "Dimethylsulfoxide in Adult Respiratory Stress Syndrome," *Annual New York Academy of Science* (1983).

Koesis, JJ, Harkaway, S, Snyder, R, "Biological Effects of the Metabolites of Dimethylsulfoxide," *Annual New York Academy of Science* (1975).

Metcalf, JW, "MS—A Dietary Derivative of DSMO," *J. Eq. Vet. Sci.* (1983).

Metcalf, JW, "MSM Status Report," *Eq. Vet. Data* (1986).

Miura K et al., "Cystine Uptake and Glutathione Level in Endothelial Cells Exposed to Oxidative Stress," *Am. Jrl. Physiol.* (1992).

Morton, JI, Siegel, BV, "Effects of Oral Dimethylsulfoxide and Dimethylsulfone on Murine Autoimmune Lymphoproliferative Disease," *Proc. Soc. Exper. Bio. Med.* (1986).

Murav ev, UV et al., "The efficacy of long-term application of dimethyl sulfoxide in a complex therapy of patients with systemic scleroderma." Institute of Pharmacology, AMS USSR, translated by Inlingua Translation Services, Princeton, NJ.

Nagasawa, H, "The In Vitro and In Vivo Effects of Dimethylsulfoxide on the Pituitary

Secretion of Growth Hormone and Prolactin in Mice," *Annual New York Academy of Science* (1983).

Oae, S and Okuyama, T, "Organic Sulfur Chemistry; Biochemical Aspects," CRC Press, Boca Raton, FL, 1992.

Pearson, TW, Dawson HJ and Lackey HB, "Natural Occurring Levels of Dimethylsulfoxide in Selected Fruits, Vegetables, Grains and Beverages," *J. Agric. Food Chem.* (1981).

Pereira, RR, Harper, WJ, Gould, IA, "Volatile Sulfur Compounds in Milk I: Effect of Chemical Form of Sulfur-35 on Selective Labeling of Milk Constituents and Free Sulfur Compounds," *J. Dairy Sci.* (1966).

Repine, JE, Fox, RB, Berger, EM, "Effect of Dimethylsulfoxide on the Bactericidal Function of Polymorphonuclear Leukocytes," *Ann. N. Y. Acad. Sci.* (1983).

Richmond, VL, "Incorporation of Methylsulfonylmethane Into Guinea Pig Serum Proteins," *Life Sciences* (1986).

Richmond, VL, "Incorporation of Methylsulfonylmethane Into Guinea Pig IgG, Transferrin and Albumin Fractions and Tissues," Pacific Northwest Research Foundation, Seattle, WA.

Robert McCabe, and Jack Remington, "Toxoplasmosis: The Time Has Come," *New England Journal of Medicine* 318 (1988).

Rodale, Jl, and Staff, *The Complete Book of Minerals for Health*, Emmaus, PA: Rodale Books, Inc., 1972.

Scherbel, AL et al., "Further observations on the effect of dimethyl sulfoxide in patients with generalized scleroderma (progressive systemic sclerosis)." *Annals New York Academy of Sciences* (1969):613–629.

Schroeder, H, *The Trace Elements and Man*, Greenwich, CT: Devin Adair, 1973.

Sehnert, KW, Clague, AF, Cheraskin, E, "Improvement in Renal Function Following EDTA Chelation and Multi-Vitamin-Trace Mineral Therapy: A Study in Creatinine Clearance," *Med Hypotheses* (1984).

Sellnow, I, "MSM—An Aid From Nature," *Canadian Horseman* (1989).

Somer, E, *The Essential Guide to Vitamins and Minerals*, NY: Harper Collins, 1995.

Tapadinhas, MJ, Rivera, IC, Bignamini, AA, "Oral Glucosamine Sulfate in the Management of Arthrosis," Report on a Multi-center Open Investigation in Portugal, (1982).

Teigland, MB and Saurino, VR, "Clinical Evaluation of Dimethylsulfoxide in Equine Applications," *Ann. N. Y. Acad. Sci.* (1975).

Vaughn, L et al., *Prevention Magazine's Complete Book of Vitamins and Minerals*, NY, NJ: Wings Books, 1994.

Ward, PA, Till GO, Kunkel R, Beauchamp, C, "Evidence for Role of Hydroxyl Radical in Complement and Neutrophil-dependent Tissue Injury," *J. Clin. Inv.* (1983).

Wilford, John Noble. "Dinosaur Theory: Sulfur Was Villain (But Hero for Humans)," *The New York Times* (1995).

Williamson, J, Boettcher, B, Meister, A, "Intracellular Cysteine Delivery System that Protects Against Toxicity by Promoting Glutathione Synthesis," *Proc. Natl. Acad. Sci.* (1982).

Vines, G, "A gut feeling (disease-causing bacteria in junk food)," *New Scientist*, 159 2146:26.

Wright, J and Littleton, K, "Defects in Sulfur Metabolism," *Intl. Clin. Nutr. Rev.* (1989).

Wright, J and Kirk, FR, "Defects in Sulfur Metabolism II: Apparant Failure of Sulphate Conjugation," *Intl. Clin. Nutr. Rev.* (1989).

Suggested Readings

Challem J, *All About Vitamins*. Garden City Park, NY: Avery Publishing, 1998.

Lieberman S and Bruning N, *The Real Vitamin and Mineral Book*, Garden City Park, NY: Avery Publishing Group, 1997.

Index

Acid/alkaline balance,
    11–12, 15, 24–25
Acne
    MSM and, 24–25
    sulfur deficiency and,
        15
Aging, 64
Allergens, 32, 33–34
Allergies
    about, 31–33
    conventional
        treatments for, 37–38
    MSM and, 36–40
    substances that cause.
        See Allergens.
    who can develop, 35
Allergy shots. See
    Allergies,
    conventional
    treatments for.
Amino acids, 17–18. See
    also Sulfur amino
    acids.
Antihistamines. See
    Allergies,
    conventional
    treatments for.
Arthritis
    conventional
        treatment for, 56–57
    glucosamine and, 57
    MSM and, 55–56
    types of, 55
Asthma, MSM and, 61

Beauty
    diet and, 29

MSM and, 21

See also Hair; Nails; Skin.

Betaine hydrochloride, 52

Biotin, 16, 28

Burns, MSM and, 61

Cancer, MSM and, 58–59

Cartilage, 56

Cells, balancing pressure of, 15

Collagen
cartilage production and, 57
importance of, 26–27
natural versus injected, 27
sulfur's effect on, 25, 27

Colon cancer, 59

Constipation
fiber and, 50
MSM and, 49

Cysteine, 18

Dermis, 26

Diabetes, MSM and, 60

Diet, sulfur in the, 14

Digestive complaints, when not to use MSM for, 52

Dimethyl sulfide (DMS), 8

Dimethylsulfoxide (DMSO), 9–11

DMS. *See* Dimethyl sulfide.

DMSO. *See* Dimethylsulfoxide.

Dust mites. *See* Mites.

Epidermis, 26

FDA. *See* Food and Drug Administration.

Fibrinogen, 16

Fibromyalgia, MSM and, 61

Food and Drug Administration (FDA), 68

Foods
mineral content of, 12

preservatives, 20
processed, 14
sulfur-rich, 13
Free radicals, 16

Glucosamine, 16, 57
Glutathione, 16

Hair, MSM and, 28
Heartburn, MSM and, 50–51
Herschler, Robert, 9
Histamines, 33
Hydrochloric acid, MSM and, 52

Immune system, allergies and, 32
Immunotherapy. *See* Allergies, conventional treatments for.
Inorganic sulfur. *See* Sulfur, inorganic.
Insulin, 16, 60

Jacob, Stanley, 9, 65, 68

Keratin, 11, 28

Ligaments, 57

Methionine, 18
Methyl-sulfonyl-methane. *See* MSM.
Minerals, 12–13
Mites, 34
MSM
    allergies and, 36–40
    anti-inflammatory, as an, 10
    arthritis and, 55–56
    asthma and, 61
    beauty and, 21
    body's need for, 64
    burns and, 61
    buying, 68
    cancer and, 58–59
    constipation and, 49
    diabetes and, 60
    dosage of,

recommended, 64–65

forms of, 66–67

hair and, 28

heartburn and, 50–51

muscle stiffness and, 58

nails and, 28

pain relief and, 54

parasites and, 43, 47–48

pets and, 69

production of, nature's, 8

safety of, 68

skin and, 22–25

supplementing with, importance of, 19

therapeutic effects, discovery of, 9

See also Sulfur.

Muscle stiffness, cause of, 58

MSM and, 58

Nails, MSM and, 28

Nonsteroidal anti-inflammatory drugs (NSAIDs), 55–57

NSAIDs. *See* Nonsteroidal anti-inflammatory drugs.

Nutrients, body's need for, 12

Osteoarthritis. *See* Arthritis.

Pain relief, MSM and, 54

Parasites

about, 42–43

conventional treatments for, 48

diagnosing infestation of, 45–46

effects of, on the body, 46–47

MSM and, 43, 47–48

transmission of, 43–45

Pets, MSM and, 69

Preservatives, food, 20

Prostaglandin, 56

Protein

amino acids and
synthesis of, 17–18

collagen and, 26

Rheumatoid arthritis. *See*
Arthritis.

Skin
elasticity of, MSM
and, 25

layers of, 25–26

MSM and, 22–25

Subcutis, 26

Sulfa drugs, 20

Sulfites, 20

Sulfur
about, 7, 11–12

compounds
dependent on, 15

deficiency of, 15

food sources of, 13, 14

inorganic, 20

See also MSM.

Sulfur amino acids,
18–19

Sweat glands, 23–24

Taurine, 18–19

Tendons, 57

Toxins, MSM and, 23

Wrinkles, MSM and, 27